PERSEPHONE

Reports on works in progress in the Medical Section at the Goetheanum

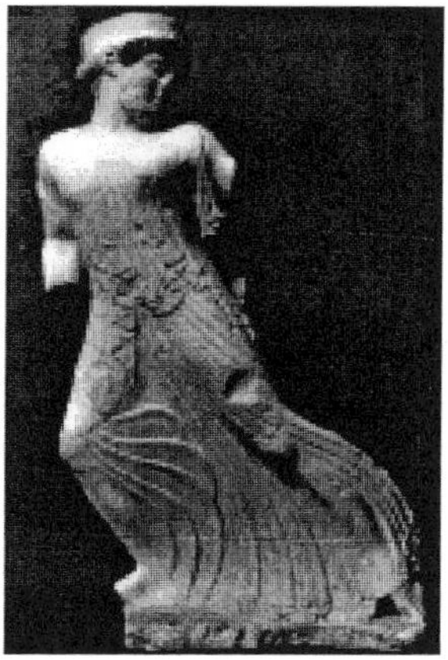

AF754461

"Entirely Soul - *Persephone*,
Entirely Human Spirit - *Demeter*"

That is how these figures appear before us in the holy drama of Eleusis.* A series of working reports by the Medical Section at the Goetheanum will be given the name Persephone, beginning with this issue. It is the soul's destiny to work its way out of earth darkness to the spirit's light. This path is associated with disease and error. If health and knowledge are to be attained, the forces of the earth's depths (Persephone in Hades) and of the heavenly heights (Persephone united with Dionysos and with her mother Demeter) need to be harmonized. We hope that the work reports and results that are published here will be helpful on this path.

* See *Genesis of Tragedy and the Sacred Drama of Eleusis*, by Edouard Schure and lecture one (August 25, 1912), in *Initiation, Eternity and The Passing Moment*, by Rudolf Steiner.

Illustration, Page One: *Persephone*

WILLEM F. DAEMS

CHELIDONIUM / CURCUMA COMP.

A Medicament-Study

Previous History, Development, Realization

Translated by Harold Jurgens

Published by the Medical Section of the School for Spiritual Science

Goetheanum, Dornach

MERCURY PRESS

Translated by Harold Jurgens from the original German
Chelidonium / Curcuma Comp, Eine Heilmittel Studie, Vorgeschichte, Entwicklung, Verwirklichung, published by Verlag am Goetheanum, which granted permission for the translation.

ISBN 0-929979-69-9

Printed and published in the United States by

MERCURY PRESS

Fellowship Community
241 Hungry Hollow Road
Spring Valley, New York 10977

I should not neglect to draw your attention to the fact that what I'm telling you here is not borrowed from old medical writings, it is based on present-day spiritual-scientific research. However, sometimes one has to try to go back to the older literature, because the newer literature hasn't yet developed a terminology for these things. But it would be a big mistake for anyone to think that what I'm telling you here is only taken from older writings.

For instance, I would never consider it to be my business to arrive at something through a study of Paracelsus, but sometimes I have an urge to see how a discovery I have made sounds in his language, that is the way I would like to ask you to receive what I'm trying to give.

RUDOLF STEINER[1]

DEDICATED TO

PHARMACIST WALTHER SCHNEIDER

DECEMBER 7, 1929 - JUNE 5, 1990

CONTENTS

Foreword - Michaela Glöckler 1

Introduction 3

Medicinal Plants Two Thousand Years Old 7

Choleodoron 10

Chelidonium - Curcuma - Cucurbita 13

Rudolf Steiner's Note: Foundation for the New Chelidonium/Curcuma Comp. Preparation 19

The "Magnetic Nature" of Curcuma 27

Notes 35

FOREWORD

About eight years ago Heribert Kaufmann from Weleda AG, Schwäbisch Gmünd and Walther Schneider from Weleda AG, Arlesheim asked Friedrich Lorenz, the leader of the Medical Section at the Goetheanum at the time, to found a circle to work with basic research problems in anthroposophical pharmaceutics. He did so.

This work was interrupted when Friedrich Lorenz died in the spring of 1987, and it was continued by me, as his successor. At the suggestion of Walther Schneider, the first medicament that we worked on was Choleodoron®, for which Rudolf Steiner had given an indication that had previously been ignored. An investigation of the underlying data led to new insights and Walter Schneider made a number of experimental preparations on this basis. In the meantime both Heribert Kaufmann and Walther Schneider had also passed over death's threshold. Willem F. Daems now began to do scientific work on the preparation that had been modified in this way and to present it to interested anthroposophical doctors and pharmacists in the form of the following article. This has given rise to an outstanding example of a monograph of an anthroposophical medicament, for which I would like to thank him heartily. Here scientific exactness is combined with a love for detail and a deep respect for the healing forces that are present in nature's processes.

We especially thank Weleda AG, Arlesheim for their financial aid for this work.

Medical Section at The Goetheanum
St. John's 1992

Michaela Glöckler

INTRODUCTION

The first medical course that Rudolf Steiner gave from March 21 to April 9, 1920 in Dornach[1] is generally regarded as the impetus that made pharmacists begin to prepare medicaments on the basis of anthroposophical knowledge. In any case, one can hardly imagine the turmoil immediately after the course as we tried to satisfy the rapidly rising flood of doctors' requests.

However, the burgeoning activity after April 1920 had already existed on a smaller scale for some time. Oskar Schmiedel (1887 - 1959) opened up his "Chemical Laboratory, Dr. Oskar Schmiedel" in Munich in 1911, with the intention of making plant colors and a few body care products and medicaments. This is when the hair oil that is still being sold by Weleda in a modified form first arose. Oskar Schmiedel also made a special incense for phantom pains.

On March 1, 1914 he moved his laboratory to Dornach at Rudolf Steiner's suggestion. A wooden barrack was built for him at the canteen that is near the Goetheanum. He continued to make hair water, hair oil, hair cream, shaving cream and other body care products, plant colors for the Goetheanum, and occasional medicaments at the request of Rudolf Steiner, Peipers, Rascher, Noll, Wegman and other doctors who were members of The Anthroposophical Society.

In 1917 Ita Wegman (1876 - 1943) had asked Adolf Hauser, a pharmacist in Zurich, to make a mistletoe preparation which Rudolf Steiner wanted for the treatment of cancer, in an injectable form (it was called Iscador)[2]. Shortly thereafter she asked Schmiedel to make a mistletoe preparation according to her specifications. When Ita Wegman moved her gynecological practice from Zurich (1917 - 1920) to Basel (1921 - 1928) the regular production of medicaments was already in full swing.

It's understandable that the "Laboratory at The Goetheanum" could not at first fill all of the doctors' many orders.

Interested doctors had been using so-called Ritter remedies since at least 1912. Marie Ritter (died 1924) was a personality who had a special gift for inventing and making medicaments, and she had graduated from a medical school. On February 12, 1908 she wrote a letter to Rudolf Steiner from Breslau and asked him how to treat cancer of the uterus and breasts. She then made mistletoe preparations for oral administration on the basis of his indications. This contact between Rudolf Steiner and Marie Ritter gave rise to the "Ritter Remedies," which were later manufactured by a pharmaceutical company in Munich and were known to doctors in the anthroposophical movement.

Marie Ritter called these remedies "photodynamic preparations"[3]. Among her 85 plant preparations is Viscum Betulae, with an indication for stomach cancer and other problems. Her trademark was an MR (Marie Ritter) monogram with two crossed branches of mistletoe.

When the International Labor (ILAG)[4], Arlesheim first opened Ritter remedies were kept in stock. ILAG's first account book contains entries for orders from Munich. Marie Ritter came to Rudolf Steiner's second medical course in April 1921[5].

The fact that Ludwig Noll (1872 - 1930) introduced numerous tried and true combinations of medicaments into the evolutionary stream of Anthroposophical Medicine and its preparation of medicaments that arose in 1920 is important for our Choleodoron® story. The sources mention Infludo (later Infludoron®), Combudoron®, Nausyn® (later Nauseodoron), Pertudoron®, Rheumadoron® and others, but they never mention Choleodoron®.

This group of medicaments was entered on the first printed remedies list in July 1921 (or shortly after the opening of The Clinical Therapeutic Institute of Der Kommende Tag, Stuttgart, October 1922," (p 22), under the category "new remedies" as a "*remedia contra . . .*" The product had also appeared "end of September 1922" and at other times on price lists as Choleodoron® or *Remedium contra cholelithiasin*. Choleodoron® became a registered trademark in Germany as "A Remedy For The Treatment of Gall Stones" on February 26, 1922. However, there is no mention of Choleodoron® or *Remedium contra cholelithiasin* on the list of remedies that was printed in Arlesheim in July 1921.

It might be interesting to quote this first information about Choleodoron® in its entirety.

Choleodoron®

Components: The preparation is made from parts of the plants Chelidonium majus and Curcuma longa. Calculated from the raw drug content it is 0.5% Chelidonium majus and 0.2% Curcuma longa.

Indication: Disturbances of the Gall Bladder function. Congestion of the bile. Diseases of the bile passages and Gall Bladder; gall stone formation. (Cholangitis, Cholecystitis, Cholelithiasis). Bilious Pneumonia.

Method of Application and Dose: 10 - 15 drops, 3 - 4 times daily.

Therapeutic Action: The resinous substance and Cholerythrin and the Curcuma's ethereal oils in this preparation enhance secretion in the mucous membranes of the stomach and small intestine, but it mainly stimulates the secretion of bile, which begins to flow better because it becomes thinner; the blood flow in the liver is also enhanced. This eliminates congestive conditions in the liver and sluggish bile flow, and the formation of concretions is avoided.

Chelidonin, alpha and beta-homochelidonine, protopine and other morphinoid alkaloids in Chelidonium have an analgesic and spasmolytic effect on the smooth muscles of the large bile passages and of the gall bladder. Unlike opiates, the alkaloids derived from Chelidonium do not have a numbing or paralyzing effect on peristalsis. (See papers by Meyer, *Archiv für experimentelle Pathologie*, 1882, Vol.29, p398; Seved Ribbing-Rumpf, *Ärztl. Rundschau*, 1896, no. 35; Iwanov: *Medizinskoje Obosrenie*, 1898, Nr. 3; *E. Merks Jahresbericht*, 1915, XXIX. Jahrgang, pp 76,79).

Note: The emphasis on the pharmacology of active ingredients and the limited number of mostly antiquated references, and especially the reference - note well - to the review "Mercks (not Merks) Annual Report!"

Medicinal Plants Two Thousand Years Old

A Thousand Years of The Chelidonium / Curcuma Combination

It was easy to prove that (Celandine) Chelidonium and (Turmeric) Curcuma were being sold as a combination at the beginning of Anthroposophical Medicine. For instance, Gehe's Codex[6] for 1919 lists the preparation Chol-ompin of Ludwig Hermann & Co., Nuremberg, that consisted of Natriumoleinicum Natriumcholeinicum, CHELIDONIUM, Boldo, CURCUMA, Thymol, and Camphor.

On searching the literature I discovered that Thomas Sydenham (1624 - 1689) recommended the following prescription for the treatment of *colica biliosa* (gall bladder colic) and colica hysterica (uterine colic) in his "*Oper Omnia Medica*"[7]: *Rx Radicis rubiae tinctorum, Radicis curcumae ana unciam unam, Chelidonii maioris cum toto, summitatum centaurii minoris ana manipulum unum*. The method of preparation is described.

I acquired a doctor's diary[8] from the 17th century a few years ago that contains a prescription with *Schelwurtz* (*Schöllkraut* = Chelidonium) and Curcuma written underneath it, and eleven other ingredients. The country doctor who wrote the prescription probably thought that the two plants belonged together for otherwise they could just as well have appeared far apart on the list of drugs.

Or was this "combination" just a coincidence?

Is there some other reason for the combination?

It might pay to look further back into the past with respect to our Choleodoron® story.

When Dioskurides[9] described a sedge cyperus (I,4) – "that is similar to ginger" he referred to "another kind of Cyperus" that grows in India and that colors the saliva yellow when chewed, and it tastes bitter. By this Dioskurides meant tumeric or Curcuma.

The yellow coloring quality of tumeric leads to its being mixed up with saffron which is also know for its ability to color things yellow (both of these were known in antiquity as leather dyes). For instance, the Persians called turmeric "stick saffron" and in drug text books in the late Middle Ages it was called "Zafarano indo" and "Croco indiaco." One of the spices listed in Song of Solomon 4:14 is Carcom = Curcuma. This spice is translated erroneously in the King James version as saffron.

However, one also gets a mix-up between turmeric and celandine fairly early, because the latter also contains a strong yellow dye. In Islamic medicine turmeric was known under the Arabic name *memith* (memithe, memitha) and as *chelidonium* in Latin contexts. The mix-up may have begun with Avicenna, the Persian doctor (980 - 1036), his Arabic word for Turmeric is *chaludumenum*, which the Latin translator made into *chelidonium*. Thus Turmeric made its way to Europe via Avicenna and Ibn Al-Baitar (died 1248). Ibn al-Baitar seems to have called the Chelidonium of Dioskurides (II, 211[10]) *curcum*; this confusion entered the drug literature in the 14th century, and it stayed there.

In a manuscript[11] by Erbario Carrarese at the end of the 14th century there is a chapter (p. 152f) on "de memithe" with the synonym "celidonia", and a chapter (p.207f) "de curcuma: with the synonym "cillidonia"! Later in 1475 a Lüneburg drug list mentions Radix Chelidonii with the synonym "Curcuma Serapionis". The Serapion - source[12] (*Sarabiyun* in Arabic) refers to the Pseudepigraphy for Ibn al-Baitar, whose drug book (*Liber aggregationis in medecinis simplicibus* in the Latin translation) has a non-existent "Serapion minor" ascribed to it.

These indications were selected because they are particularly appropriate to our theme, but many more could be cited. However, they might suffice to get someone to write a dissertation or other thorough study on "The paired medicinal plants Chelidonium/Curcuma – accidental or intentional?"

Jaundice is the main indication for turmeric in ancient texts. However it was of more importance as a spice and a dye (for leather ware, etc.). As the Dutch botanist Rembert Dodoens[13] (1516 - 1585) put it, "it's used more by painters and alchemists than for diseases."

In his dissertation on *curcuma officinarum* (the druggists turmeric) in 1748, Carl Christian Loeber[14] lists the effects on the liver and bile: Turmeric eliminates congestions in the bile ducts and liver, and removes pathogenic substances that cause cramps, enhances blood circulation, increases secretion of bile, and drives stones out of the bile ducts, the gall bladder and the ductus choledochus.

Turmeric is most effective in powder form at a dose of 1.25 - 3.5 gm; decoctions and infusions can also be used, but essences and tinctures are relatively ineffective.

Turmeric was practically forgotten in the 19th century, but systematic research in the Dutch Colonial Institute from about 1900 on, clarified a large number of questions and began a Renaissance for Curcuma in medicine.

CHOLEODORON®

From The Combination To The Composition

Just for argument's sake let us look upon the inclusion of Choleodoron® in the group of "New Remedies...which arose from spiritual scientific research" as something that wasn't reflected upon sufficiently, and let's assume that Rudolf Steiner tolerantly accepted the mixture Chelidonium/ Curcuma as a tried and true remedy.

1. In any case, an idea of Rudolf Steiner's entered into the very first stage of the manufacture that certainly was intended to bring about a qualitative improvement.

Shortly after the first medical course–in the summer of 1920–Rudolf Steiner had a conversation with Ludwig Noll (and possibly others) about the making of Iscador, a mistletoe preparation, with the aid of a centrifuge to mix it. After this Rudolf Steiner indicated that "the same procedure can also be used for the other preparations, e.g. the roots of celandine and turmeric." A more exact indication followed including the making of different Choleodoron preparations for gall bladder disorders that had existed for a shorter or longer time.

Ludwig Noll dictated this indication to Oskar Schmiedel in July 1921.

Of course the proper equipment for this was not yet available and it took until 1951 before a mixing centrifuge was constructed in accordance with Theodor Schwenk's design.

Dietrich Boie[15] gave the first, detailed report about experiences with centrifuged Choleodoron in 1970.

The medicament is still listed as Chelidonium/Curcuma praeparatum (Weleda); the response from Anthroposophical doctors has never been very great.

2. The discovery of a page from one of Rudolf Steiner's notebooks is of greater importance, for it adds a completely new conception of the preparation to its use for "Ailments of the gall bladder." The note was written about the same time (summer 1920) as a note about mistletoe on the back side of this same loose leaf page. This reverse side was published by me in 1988[16]. The first reproduction of the "Choleodoron note" follows with the permission of the administrator of Rudolf Steiner's literary estate.

Gall Bladder diseases:

Celandine - Root.

Cucurbita = retarded growth.

Intestines.

Turmeric = magnetic nature.

Boie knew about this note, because he referred to it in his Choleodoron® study, and he said that the loose leaf note indicates the use of "Cucurbita" as an additional component of the remedy. Boie didn't go into this and as far as I know no one else has either.

The new component "Cucurbita" in between celandine and tumeric is in fact the first new thing that one notices. Rudolf Steiner uses the Austrian *Scheelkraut* instead of *Schöllkraut*, so that tells us where he came from (*Schöll* is derived from Chelidonium and *Scheel* is similar to *Schiel-en* = squinting, which indicates its use as an ocular remedy)[17]. It appears important to him to emphasize the root, he underlined "root" three times, whereas otherwise Steiner was giving indications for Celandine flowers during the twenties.

What is harder to figure out is the "magnetic nature" in connection with Turmeric.

An intensive study of this page by doctors and Weleda pharmacists at the Medical Section of the School for Spiritual Science led to a consensus in making the new preparation *Chelidonium/Curcuma Comp.* The former combination, going back to antiquity became a composition that can rightly be grouped with the preparations that came from Rudolf Steiner's spiritual scientific research.

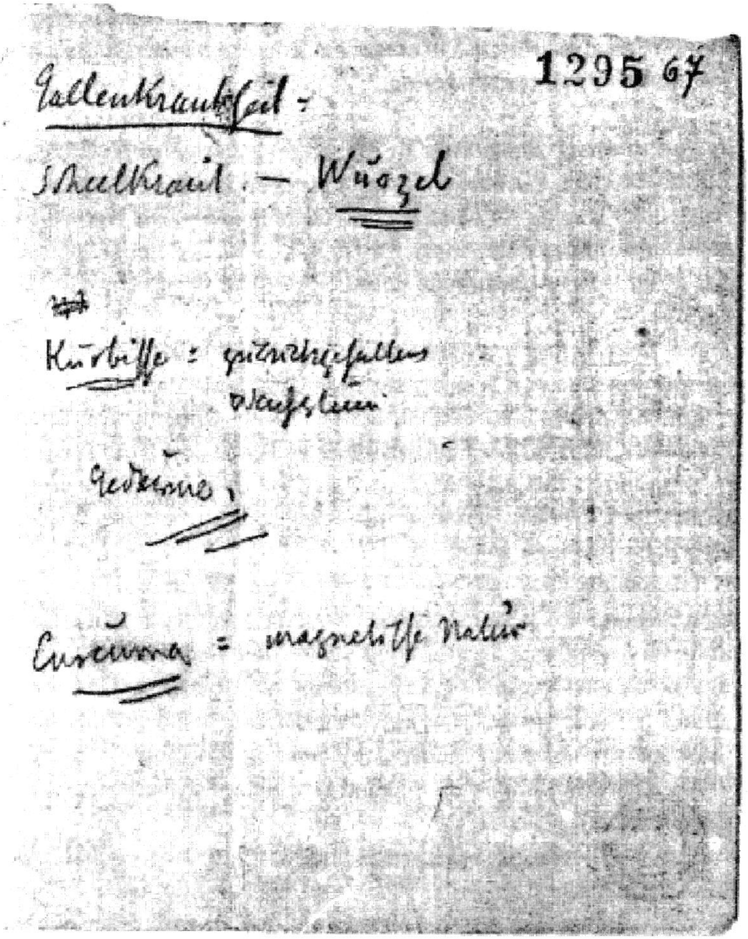
1295 67

Gallenkrankheit =

Schellkraut – Wurzel

Kürbisse = zurückgehaltenes Wachstum

Gedärme,

Curcuma = magnetische Natur

Translation of text:

Gallbladder disease

Chelidonium - root

pumpkins = retarded growth

intestines

curcuma = magnetic nature

CHELIDONIUM - CURCUMA CUCURBITA

Pharmacographic Notes on the Three Components

Chelidonium

Chelidonium majus (Linn.) or greater Celandine[18], unlike lesser celandine, belongs to the poppy family (papaveraceae).

The plant has spread like a weed all over Europe, Asia and North America. It gets to be about 2½ ft. high (1-4 ft. range) and it typically has pinnate leaves, light green above, bluish green underneath, and irregularly branched stems. The yellow flowers with four petals and four sepals pass over into vertical, long pods, containing brownish black seeds, which ants like to eat and disseminate. The herb arises from a reddish brown root stock with several heads, short and about ½ inch thick, spongy to fibrous, bearing fine rootlets and vestigial leaves.

The entire plant is permeated by a bitter juice with a disagreeable smell. In the roots the yellowish, milky sap becomes orange red.

It contains about 20 alkaloids of the protopine, protoberberine and benzophenanthridine-type. The alkaloid content in the leaves is about 0.6% (*Deutsches Arznei Buch*[9]), and in the roots it can be as much as 2%.

Chelidonine is one of the main alkaloids and it is used to standardize mono-preparations. Berberine gives the juice its yellow color. The juice contains proteolytic enzymes and has been used to treat warts externally. Other alkaloids in it are Chelerythrine, Sanguinarine and Coptisine.

Its range of effects is mainly dependent on its alkaloids. Chelidonine has a spasmolytic, musculotropic effect that is not quite as strong as that of the papaverine in opium poppy (*Papaver somniferum*). The spasmolytic effect is supported by a slightly centralizing, analgesic one. Its choleretic effect is ascribed to berberine. Sanguinarine has an inhibitory effect on the action of acetylcholinesterase.

One finds the following range of indications in the older literature:

For disorders of the liver, gall bladder, kidneys and bladder and their side effects, such as jaundice (the result of liver congestion), and edema.

Present day Chelidonium preparations with standardized Chelidonine contents are used for biliary and gastro-intestinal colics, and for cholecystitis.

Curcuma

Natives of Java and other parts of Indonesia used to do a lively trade in turmeric as spice and medicine in the first decades of the 20th century. They sold a number of turmeric species that are difficult to tell apart under the name of Temu Lawak (yellow root), so that a systematic investigation[19] became necessary to distinguish the medical turmeric from the spice variety (see p. 9 of the dissertation).

Turmeric species belong to the tropical ginger family (Zingiberaceae). The family includes typical spices and medicinal plants, like Ginger, Galanga, Zedoary, Cardamom, Melegueta and Kaempferia. They all have the chemotaxonomic marks of an extensive development of ethereal oil cells and very acrid, spicy substances.

1. The origin of medicinal turmeric is *Curcuma xanthorrhiza* Roxburgh, the Javanese yellow root.

Its rhizome is much bigger than its yellow inflorescence. Growers often remove the flowers in order to enhance the rhizome formation. The long stemmed, lanceolate leaves that grow out of the ground can get up to 40 inches long.

The habitus of the tuberous main rhizome and the long accessory rhizomes is almost identical with that of tumeric spice plants. The tuberous form, main rhizome is the drug that is traded, - *Rhizoma Curcumae javanicae.* The commodity comes onto the market peeled, cut into thin slices and dried at ca. 50°C.

Turmeric root smells something like ginger; it has a bitter taste and it colors saliva yellow.

Medicinal Turmeric contains 5 - 8% ethereal oil. The mixture of yellow pigments is called curcumin. Curcurmins are Diarylheptanoids, - mainly Diferuloylmethane and its derivatives. The curcumin content is usually around 1% (see below).

All ethereal oils have a broad range of physiological effects, but the carminative and choleretic ones predominate here. The oil also has a fungitoxic effect.

The curcumins and the ethereal oil are responsible for the choleretic, cholekinetic and anti-inflammatory effects. Recent investigations indicate the presence of antimutagenic properties in curcumine.

2. Turmeric spice comes from the yellow root of *Curcuma domestica Valeton* (= C. longa Koenig non L.).

There are two main kinds:

- *longa*, cylindrically compressed, finger-shaped accessory rhizomes 1½ x 5/8 inches. The "longa" commodity is turmeric spice;
- *rotunda*, bulbous main rhizome 1½ x 1¼ inches; which is used for reproduction.

The "longa" rhizome is cooked for an hour or treated with hot water, whereby the bulb's reserve starch conglutinates. Then the tubers are dried on mats in the sun.

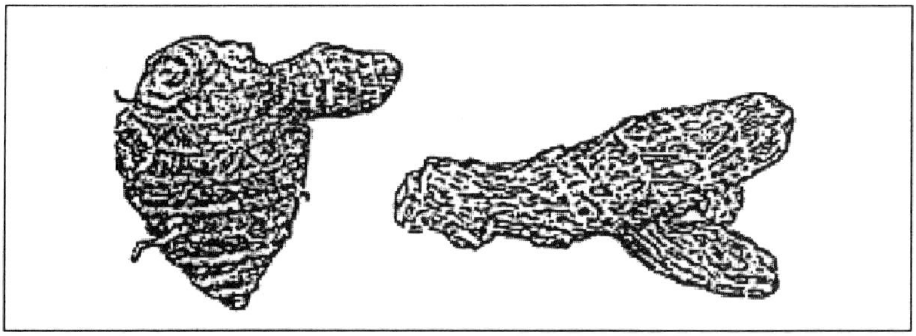

The tuberous main rhizome and digitiform accessory one of Curcuma domestica (from Gassner).

See previous page for ingredients and sphere of activity. A chemical analysis of the two species gives a clear-cut distinction between them:

Turmeric Spice	*1.5% Ethereal Oil., up to 3% Curcumin*
Medicinal Turmeric	*5-8% Ethereal Oil, approx. 1% Curcumin*

The ethereal oil of medicinal turmeric contains about 5% dimethyl benzyl alcohol (which may be something that is created during the distillation); this substance is absent in the spice's oil. On the other hand, the curcumin mixture of turmeric spice contains bisdesmethoxycurcumin, which inhibits choleresis, and was also found in the oil of medicinal turmeric.

One can easily identify the two kinds with a simple color reaction.

The physiological and therapeutic effects of the two varieties of turmeric overlap. The curcumins have a choleretic effect, and the essential oils have a cholekinetic and anti-inflammatory effect.

According to Hager[20] therapists have had good results with turmeric in patients with cholelithiasis, cholecystitis, cholangitis and injuries to the liver's parenchyma.

Cucurbita

The third component in Rudolf Steiner's note is "Cucurbita" - and for this we chose *Cucurbita maxima*, giant squash.

Bryony is a cucurbita, and it is an important remedy in anthroposophically extended medicine. Luffa and Bryony are also used in homeopathy. Cucurbita seeds are the foundation in preparations for the treatment of enlarged prostrate glands. But otherwise cucurbita are hardly used in medicine anymore. In the early part of this century Colocynth (*Citrullus colocynthis*), squirting cucumber (*Ecballium elaterium*) and Momordica species were still recommended.

Homeopathic doses of pumpkin seeds have been used for severe nausea or explosive vomiting immediately after meals, that sometimes accompanies gastrointestinal disorders[21].

In the strict sense of the term, "Cucurbita" covers a large variety of species in the Cucumis and Cucurbita families. Some of the best known are:

Pumpkin, *Cucurbita pepo*
Giant squash, *Cucurbita maxima*
Cucumber, *Cucumis sativus*
Muskmelon, *Cucumis melo*
Watermelon, *Citrullus lanatus*
Colocynth, *Citrullus colocynthis*
Bottle gourd, *Cucurbita lagenaria*
Squirting Cucumber, *Ecbollium elaterium*

Cucurbita maxima Duchesne, giant or eating squash is the cucurbita species and variety that furnishes the pulp mass for the new Chelidonium/ Curcuma Comp. Giant squash is the right name for it, because its fruits can weigh as much as 220 lbs.

Cucurbita generally have the following distinguishing marks:

- very little root growth;
- large leaves attached to creeping stems which sometimes climb up things with mostly forked tendrils,
- large, often yellow flowers, and small, medium or enormous fruits which botanists look upon as true berries with shells.

The pulp inside is 95% or more water, and the remainder consists of minerals, vitamins and aromatic substances. Even though the huge, watery body only consists of 2.5 - 5% solid substances, it can still give an "organized" semisolid or toughly solid impression.

These berries are converted into thirst quenchers, marmalades, sauces, etc., but we won't go into their useful character here.

Rudolf Steiner's Note

The Foundation for the New Chelidonium / Curcuma Comp. Preparation

After studying Rudolf Steiner's so-called pharmaceutical, medical note books for years we arrived at new insights into his way of working. The discovery that some of the notes arose after Rudolf Steiner consulted the older literature – and he had a large number of such books in his library – led to a fundamentally new view of these notes' importance. Rudolf Steiner worked like any other scientist does here, he briefly summarized things he had read, from memory, so that the formulations are often just like they were in the text books.

Thus with some of these notes one can ask oneself whether a remedy stood in the background, and whether one can really speak of a "prescription." For one cannot find a single prescription among these notes that indicates the amounts, preparation time, auxiliary substances and form of the medicament.

Another question one can ask is,– if the notes were supposed to give an idea about medicaments, why didn't Rudolf Steiner immediately give them to the pharmacists who were there, or why didn't he feed his views into the daily lab work? That he didn't do this is shown by the fact that many notes did not get into the Weleda archives, but were only found much later in his literary estate.

That was the starting situation for the Choleodoron note.[22] It was discovered on the reverse side of a mistletoe note through a search for indications on how to make mistletoe preparations. (see Above)

The new, third component "Cucurbits" strikes one's attention right away when one looks at the note, and by association one immediately gets a fundamental concept for the invention and preparation of remedies that is in line with spiritual science. The concept is based on the following elements:

- *Health* is the continual striving to create and maintain an equilibrium between two physiological systems that are at odds with each other, or to preserve the sound totality in the middle;
- *Disease* is the loss of this healthy middle; it's disruption of the equilibrium;
- *Healing* is the result of an effort to recover the lost center;
- *A healing agent or medicament* is any instrument that restores the soundness or health in the middle.

On this basis polar processes in nature can become remedies for human processes that have fallen out of the middle, and are therefore pathological. The polar healing forces of nature need a connecting link in order to reach the disturbed center, regardless of which physiological region it is in. This can only be found in a third, mediating natural substance and/or in an adequate pharmaceutical process. A real, remedial composition can arise on this basis. Such a composition is a real work of art and a mercurial agent that makes its healing power effective towards both poles.

For instance, according to this concept of Rudolf Steiner's, the following are works of art:

- *Cardiodoron.* Polarity of European primula and Scotch thistle with Henbane as the middle that is also supported by the digestion process;
- *Digestodoron.* Polarity of Ferns and Willows that is enhanced in the connecting middle by digestion there;
- *Hepatodoron.* Polarity of Strawberry and Grape leaves; the ends are connected by a special pharmaceutical method.

Chelidonium / Curcuma

One can easily see the polarity– Celandine / turmeric – and the middle –cucurbits – from the way they are arranged on Steiner's note page.

If one studies Pelikan's[23] excellent description of the nature of Chelidonium and Curcuma and if one adds one's own observations and knowledge to this, it is obvious that in the polarity that becomes effective here, Celandine is the salt principle and turmeric is the sulfur principle.

The strong formation of alkaloids and the mighty root structure[24] (See sketch of it below) in Celandine contributes to the salt classification, whereas turmeric is practically nothing but a rhizome (See photo below) that is overpowered by the sulfuric forces in the flowers (essential oils and dyes.)

Cucurbits

The cucurbits are a new and unusual element in the composition. There is a small monograph[25] on Cucumbers, Melons and Cucurbits in Rudolf Steiner's private library, which may have oriented him about Cucurbits in general. Cucurbits cannot raise themselves above the ground, in spite of their great growing power; their "retarded growth" (see note) is an obvious, natural process. Rudolf Steiner no doubt connected the latter with the retarded growth in the realm of liver and bile processes.

Plants develop their manifold nature and variety of shapes with the cooperation of all seven planets. However, the sun's influence on Cucurbits is weak – they can't stand up – and so is the moon's influence – they have hardly any roots. The predominant characteristic of cucurbits is their fruity formation as a swelling of spherical or otherwise rounded, juicy berries – the result of the purest Mercury effect.

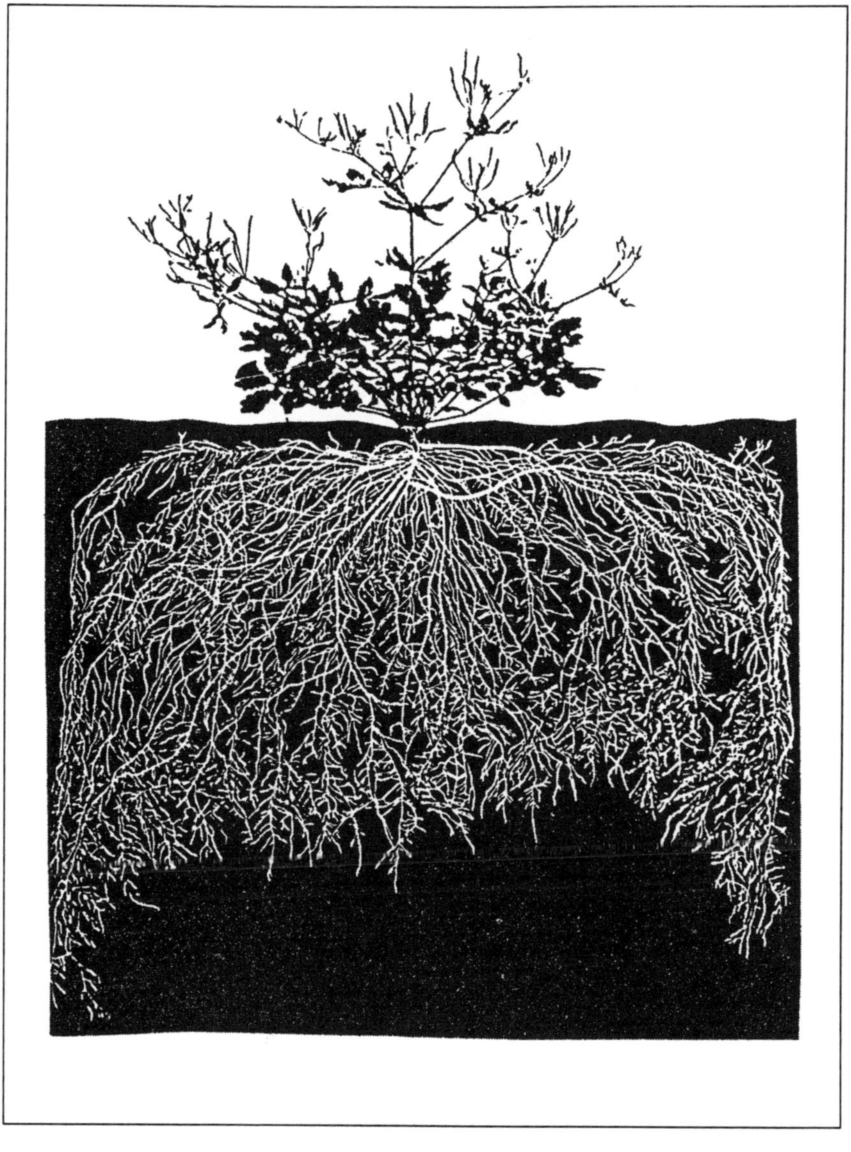

Celandine, Chelidonium majus Linn.
The root region of a single plant

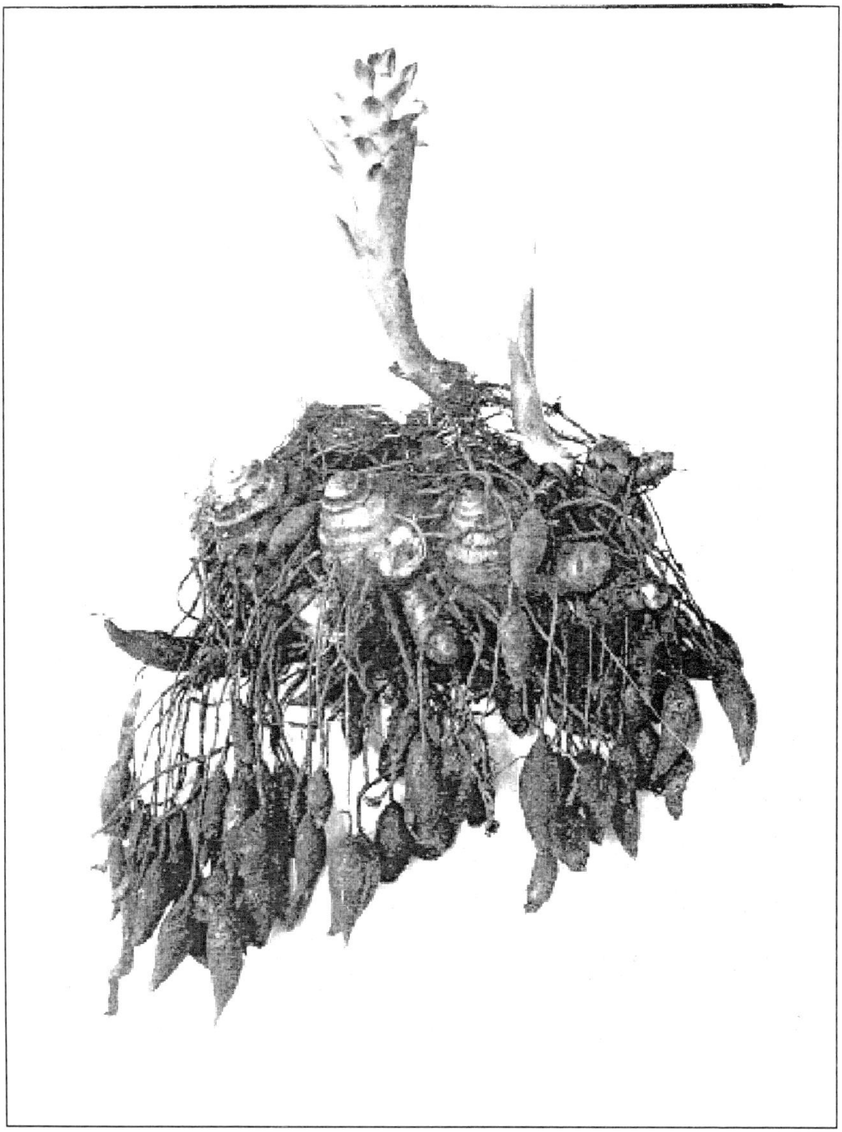

Turmeric
Curcuma xanthorrhiza (photo)

A brief discussion of Galen's (2nd Century A.D.) theories follow[26]

People in past millennia lacked our extraordinary knowledge of active ingredients, among other things, but anyone who can only snicker at their achievements should consider that their admiral power of observation and tested, practical experience, gave them a better grasp of the integral quality of nature's raw materials (as food stuffs and remedies), than we have today with our chemical, physical data. The characterizations in the Galenian system of grades or degrees can still help us today, in spite of its somewhat decadent and schematic character.

In the Middle Ages drugs were listed and given certain grades in accordance with their primary qualities. Thus in Erbario Carrarese's manuscript mentioned above[11] we find the following qualitative stages for the plants in the new Chelidonium/Curcuma Cucurbita composition:

- *Celandine* is cold and dry in the second degree – which assigns it to the earth element.
- *Turmeric* is hot and dry in the third degree, and therefore almost as fiery as pepper, which is hot and dry at the fourth level (five element);
- *Cucurbits* (melons, cucumbers, squash, pumpkins) are put into the cold and moist category (water) at the second level.

Fire	Hot and Dry	*Turmeric*
Air	Warm and Moist	
Water	Moist and Cold	*Cucurbits*
Earth	Cold and Dry	*Celandine*

One could hardly get a clearer idea of the polarity and middle for this composition.

Cucurbits can give one an instructive example of polarity as a primal phenomenon[27] Of course the primal phenomenon of polarity is already germinally present in every cell. If one cuts a pickled cucumber at right angles to its long axis, one sees a distinct separation between two kinds of tissues, - a firmer white one, and a fluidie, glassy one. If the cut is made at the stem's end (earth pole) one sees the solid, white figure at the center as an earthly element surrounded by a peripherally determined, glassy, sunny sheathe-formation. If the cut is at the opposite flower pole the situation is reversed,– the glassy part lies in the midst of a firm, white sheathe. This is an image of earthy, saline effects and sunny, sulfuric ones.

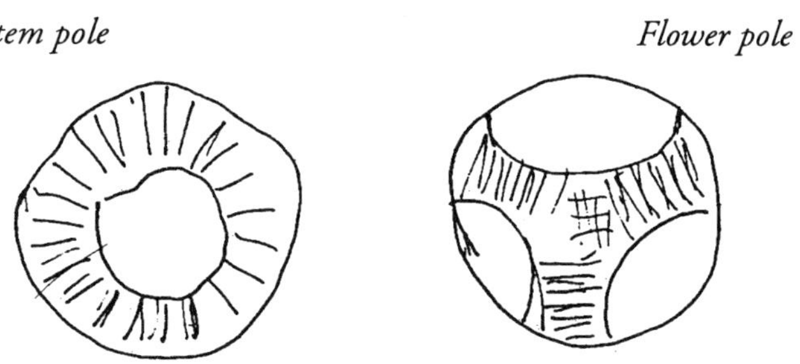

The shaded parts are glassy

All of the original, wild kinds, of cucurbits were permeated by toxic substances that had drastic effects; our recent, cultivated forms are free of this and they are all more or less sweet.

These bitter substances are tetracyclic terpenes that are connected in a glycosidic manner and are accompanied by enzymasen that can cleave them. One calls them cucurbitacins; 14 of them (ABC...N) have been isolated.

The range of effects of these bitter principles goes from a toxic effect (vomiting) to a mild laxative, diuretic and digestive effect via a drastic purging effect.

Therewith we have arrived at the "intestines" on Rudolf Steiner's note.

We only know of two places where Rudolf Steiner indicated the use of melons in therapy[28]:

1. He recommended "melons internally" for a woman who had a "digestive disorder and jaundice, in the fall of 1912."[29]

2. He described the beginning of arteriosclerosis, "The same process begins if one accustoms a patient to do without melons, and then gives him the same in a low potency as a remedy. I have often recommended it when there was only the very first indication of arteriosclerosis. Melons work in a more inner way whereas birch leaf tea has a strong effect. If I had an institution I would supplement the dinners of people who were in danger of getting arteriosclerosis with a slice of melon every three weeks." [29]

I can't resist referring to two "intestinal" passages in Walahfrid Strabos "Hortulus" [30].

(He was an abbot on Reichenau Island in Lake Constance, in the 19th Century). The first one is verses 143 - 146 in the chapter on gourds, pumpkins and squashes; it is about *viscera ventris* in the Latin original. The second four verses (177 - 180) are about melons; here again he is talking about *viscera:*

(143 - 146) However, if one lets the fruit endure the summer's heat on the vine until it is ripe, and then cuts the vicera out of its bulging body, it can be shaped into a vessel for everyday use.

(177 - 180) Garden delicacies. For the white flesh and aroma are tasty to the gums, and such food will not insult the hard molars; when chewed and swallowed rapidly its natural forces keep the body's intestines cool.

The "Magnetic Nature" of Turmeric

Anyone who saw the "Magnetic Nature" in reference to turmeric in Rudolf Steiner's note must have wondered what that was all about. It could be that this is why it took so long for the note to be elaborated.

However, anyone who studies the life and work of Theophrastus von Hohenheim (1493 - 1541), known as Paracelsus from 1529 on, and who tries to piece together his numerous remarks about magnetism, will find a solution for the "Magnetic Nature" of a plant or drug in the work of this genial medical theologian of the Renaissance.

One cannot fail to recognize the effect that Paracelsus' work had upon Anthroposophy and Anthroposophical medicine. According to Rudolf Steiner,[31] Paracelsus is "someone who comes very close to Anthroposophical views." Out of a certain overview of the respective connections one can rightly say that Paracelsus' art of healing is Anthroposophical medicine at the time of the late Renaissance.

An introduction to the theme "Magnetism in the Therapy Systems of Previous Centuries" would be necessary to really clarify the problem. However, even if such descriptions were kept very brief, they would take up too much space in the framework of our information about one composition. I will therefore limit myself to one preliminary idea, a number of quotes from Paracelsus, and a summary at the end.

Paracelsus was not the first to reject Hippocratism and Galenism for Renaissance medicine, with torrents of abuse. One of his predecessors was Nicholas of Poland, a native of Germany who had studied in Dominican schools and who then made a name for himself in Cracow in the last third of the 13th century[32].

Nicholas attacked the medical tradition of the Arabs and Scholastics very sharply in his "Antipocras". He put practice above theories, as Paracelsus did later. For him the healing power of a medicament is based on *virtus caelestica* (heavenly virtue) that is held fast in the remedy as *virtus occulta* (hidden force) with the aid of *virtus astrigena* "Astral mediation or power of the astral world". Nicholas assumes that such medicines that are filled with *virtutes occultae* work from outside and pull diseases out of the body, somewhat as a magnet does.

Now let us listen to what Parcelsus says in Sudhoff's edition of his complete works.[33, 34]

The texts that have been selected should make it possible to get an idea of Paracelsus' views about "magnetic force."

The following definition is in the short chapter on Precious Stone, in Paracelsus' "Coellum philosophorum;"[35] "A magnet is an iron stone, for it pulls iron towards it."

Sudhoff dates the Hohenheimer's earliest writings at about 1420. There he already describes "magnetic force" as a sympathy-phenomenon, and that that also applies to eating and drinking; [36] "The four elements that shall give men their fruits are preserved by the outside world. We want to discuss how things are maintained. In the same way that a man has to eat and drink in order to remain the way that he was created; for he has grown in a way that is less perfect than the way others grow. Just as eating and drinking is visible, so his other members draw things down to themselves from it. For that is the magnetic force of which we have an example in a magnet, already for the reason that it attracts visible things through an invisible force, so it forms our members in our body and makes them attract the things that sustains them. For it's not only the stomach, – every (member) is fed in an invisible way like the stomach, which later is fed in a visible way. A doctor should know something about the invisible."

In his paper on Algae [37] Paracelsus says that a medicinal plant can act like a magnet and not like an astringent such as Persicoria; "So I also wanted to tell you that this plant, when taken after influenza can have a wonder effect on somebody, even if it isn't green, but withered, or burned, distilled and extracted as water, oil and alkali salts. However, it doesn't work in a magnetic way, – it does everything through an ordinary application."

So he is telling us that one doesn't apply algae in a magnetic way, but in the usual, normal way.

The manner in which honey takes its sweetness from the earth, is compared with a magnet's power of attraction.[38] "In order to describe the nature and character of honey we should first understand that the primary material in honey is in the earth's sweetness, which is placed on plants in nature and is attracted by them through the magnetic property of these plants."

Paracelsus knew magnets in the form of magnetic iron (stones), and also as permanent magnets, which are both the "materialistic" kind. He must have seen right from the beginning that healing forces and other kinds of forces in the universe are related or comparable to *vis attractiva magnetis,* the magnet's power of attraction. In his "De Meteoris" [39] he says the following about this, after he described the meteors that fall on the earth; "For that stones are attracted is not nature's doing, and they are like nothing in it, for they are fixed and remain lying on the ground. But one can't deny that iron is related to them when a magnet attracts them; so its good to remember that these are also magnets in the heavens which do what we said, and one can find them in nature."

We have a "heavenly magnet" in us,[40] "O you doubting fellow and Peter of little faith, you who let yourself by swayed by every wind and who sink so easily. You've to blame for that through your despairing faith which is so weak and small in you; your sensual, evil thoughts bring you to that point and inflict such things upon you. You have a magnet hidden in you for that, so that you attract such things. That is the heavenly magnet above all the other magnets that pick up iron and steel or attract them. It's also above the essential quintessence or stellar magnets that discover fallen and concealed iron. The heavenly magnet is so powerful when it becomes exhalted, that it draws anything it wants out of the four elements from a hundred or thousand miles away. I will tell you some more about this and completely satisfy you with the two marvelous examples that follow."

Paracelsus described the healing power of the Pfäfer baths in a wonderful way in 1535.[41]

Chemical analyses have shown that the waters of Bad Pfäfer have very few minerals in them. Paracelsus felt that it was elemental water or excellent water and therefore he didn't think it could be looked at from the view point of the Three Principles, (Salt, Mercury and Sulfur). He ascribed its healing effect to its inherent Vis attractiva magnetis; "This bath's attack on diseases is brought about in two ways, - through the drawing out of the materials from which the disease comes, and through the destruction of the same. Such examples indicate this. Just as God gave magnets the power to attract iron, so he also gave the Pfäfer water the power to draw all of the diseases that are know to doctors out of a sick body; that is the recommended wound medicine. That water is the medicine that doctors should use for all hopeless diseases. That's like saying that this bath will heal where other natural effects won't. If someone asks why, the magnetic force will testify."

Paracelsus often used the direct power of "magnes" or magnetized iron. He prescribed numerous mixtures of medicaments with pulverized magnes for internal use. And of course he used magnets in surgery to remove foreign bodies with iron in them. [42] "People also say that there are roots and herbs that can open locks. That's ridiculous, for something like that has never been demonstrated. There's also a lot of talk about precious stones that can pull out things in a wound, and that no nail is pounded in so far that it can't be pulled out by them, but it's foolish of them to believe it. Herbalists are quite impressed by such tales. A lot of this talk is so much hot air. Herbs' power to draw is like that of a magnet and namely like this, – the latter will attract iron that is loose and unencumbered, but not iron that is attached or elevated. The same applies to herbs, but no more than that. But that various locks were opened or that nails were pulled out of walls, – that occurred through magicians who compared the magnet of the earth with the magnet of the firmament and thereby also pulled nails out of walls, raised latches on doors and pulled locks behind them after this or that magnet. Even barbed arrows have been pulled out with such magnets. Likewise various roots and herbs that have the power to attract were connected with the stars in heaven by magicians, and then they could pull things out just like the magnets just mentioned. But this doesn't mean that any root can do this, or that any magnet can do it. Also they degenerate after awhile, die off and disintegrate, for death is in all things." Thus even herbs and roots can have a magnetic power of attraction. The passage just cited has brought us into the realm of magic practices.[43] Let's also take a look at his treatment of lumbago, because I think that this will enable us to understand the "magnetic nature" of turmeric.

First we have a description of lumbago (Hexenschuss="witch's shot" in German) as a real shot of a witch[44] :"Then we also have lumbago, as the shots of witches and magicians are called, when they injure a man or give him a hump when they magically introduce ashed, hair, feathers, pigs' bristles, fish bones or many other strange things into his foot or into some other part of the body without breaking the skin.

"Without opening the skin! - and now this shot has to be brought out through the skin again[45] : "But it's necessary to bring about a cure here, and one has to see how one can draw the shot out without opening the skin, or can drive it away without hurting the man. Here it is very necessary to pay attention and learn, and to not imitate the doctors who cut open the painful spot with shearing knives, and go deep in until they've found the hair or shot, and thereby give the man many intolerable days of pain, so that they've maltreated him like a hangman and sometimes have even killed him."

That's the way his doctor colleagues did things. So what action does Paracelsus recommend? [46]

"In order to proceed so that no cutting, burning other painful opening is required and so that one can pull things out and drive them away without worries, effort or any pain to the man, one should note that it has to be done with the magnets that attract magical things and witchcraft, namely with oak leaves, chelidonia, azoth and pulverized corals. Each of these is bound around the center by itself in the proper order, and in four and twenty hours they draw out all materials that have been shot in, so that one finds them lying outside."

Oak leaves, celandine, azoth (a well know problem), powdered coral, each according to their specific healing power, are tied to the center of the disorder, to the pathogenic thing. That's how a doctor makes use of the magnetic nature of a medicament.

Concluding Remarks

One would have to make an intensive study of everything that Paracelsus said about magnetism to be able to assess all the shades of this phenomenon's significance[48]. After going through well over a hundred magnet passages in his work one could arrive at the conclusion that "magnetic force" is a universal phenomenon in developing and finished nature (macrocosm) and in the human being (microcosm) for him. Pagel speaks[49] of a "general pattern illustrating the action of remedies which, as Paracelsus said 'attract' the agents of diseases."

The microcosmic magnet helps in this action, for the magnet in men is in constant touch with the heavenly, macrocosmic one, and it is not just a copy of it and of the heavens. Paracelsus used a very simple analogy to explain this, - just as the sun can shine through glass, and as fire can make itself noticeable through an oven's walls, so bodies can send out invisible forces[50] while they remain at rest.

This magnetic force is a "live force," Paracelsus is good with words, and here he is forming the adjective from the moon "life-force" via the genitive "force of life;" this is nothing else than the common man's expression for vis attractiva magnetis!

From the ten quotes given above one should be able to get an idea of which sphere Rudolf Steiner may have been moving in when he wrote "magnetic nature" after Curcuma on his note pad.

Turmeric's pharmodynamics is at work in the realm of Choleresis or bile formation in the liver, and in cholekinesis or the flow of bile towards the gall bladder. If the healthy equilibrium has been disturbed here, turmeric can restore it, or it can "pull well-being back into the center."

Can one ascribe this healing effect to the "magnetic nature of turmeric?"

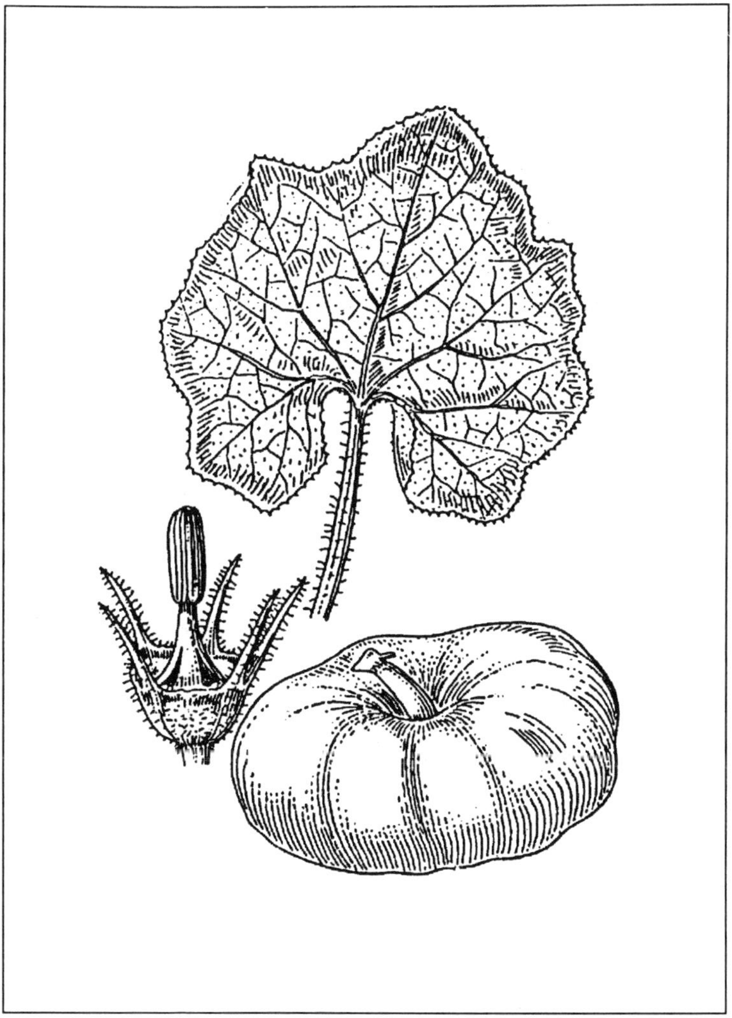

Cucurbita maxima [47]

Notes

* Compare: The Sacred Drama of Eleusis by Edouard Schure in Sacred Places of the Orient, Stuttgart [2] 1991, and Rudolf Steiner, lecture of August 25, 1912, in GA 138, Dornach [4] 1986

1 Rudolf Steiner, Spiritual Science and Medicine, twenty lectures for doctors and medical students, Dornach, March 21, 1920 (GA 312).

2 Willem F.Daems, Ita Wegman. Zürcher Zeit 1906-1920. Erste ärztliche Krebsbehandlung mit der Mistel. Mit einem Aufsatz von Ita Wegman (Weleda Schriftenreihe 17). (Ita Wegman, Zurich period 1906-1920. First treatment by a physician of cancer with mistletoe. With an essay by Ita Wegman.) Dornach: Verlag am Goetheanum 1986

3 Marie Ritter, Anleitung zum praktischen Gebrauch von Marie Ritters photodynamischen Heilmitteln. (Instructions for practical use of Marie Ritters photodynamic remedies) Breslau [1], 1912; München [3], 1915; Stuttgart [5] 1921; Innsbruck [8], 1931

4 I am not concerning myself with the early stages of ILAG (Der Kommende Tag AG; Futurum AG) (These were economic ventures attempted by various people connected with anthroposophy.)

5 Rudolf Steiner speaks of her and her remedies in the first medical course, GA 312 (Spiritual Science and Medicine), lectures 4 and 11, and in the Agriculture Course, lecture 5, GA 327

6 Gehes Codex (Special medicines index), Dresden 1919

7 Thomas Sydenham, Opera omnia medica, Patavinii 1725

8 Diarium chirurgicam (of Gottfrid Renner), 1699, p. 122

9 J. Berendes, Pedanios' Dioskurides, from Anazarbos' Pharmacology in five books. Stuttgart 1902 (Reprint: Darmstadt 1970)

10 Dioskurides (IL 4): Peri chelidonion megalon. "The juice is of the color of safran." "Drinking the root with anis and white wine, heals jaundice."

11 G. Ineichen, Die paduanische Mundart am Ende des 14. Jhts auf Grund des Erbario Carrarese. (Paduanic dialect at the end of the 14th century based on Erbario Carrarese. In: Ztschr. f. romanische Philologie, (Tübingen) 73 (1975), 38-123

12 Manfred Uhlmann, Die Medizin im Islam (Handbuch der Orientalistik, Section. 1, Suppl. Vol. VI, first paragraph). Leiden 1970, p. 283

13 Rembert(us) Dodoens, Cruyde boeck. Antwerpen 1563

14 Carl Christian Loeber, Dissertatio de curcuma officinarum eiusque genuinis virtutibus. Halle 1748

15 Dietrich Boie, Die Arzneimittelmischung in der Mischzentrifuge - Therapeutische Erfahrungen mit einem neuen Choleodoron Präparat. (Remedy mixing in a mixing centrifuge - Therapeutic experiences with a new Choleodoron preparation) Beiträge z. Erw. d. Heilkunst (Stuttgart) 23 (1970), 52-61, 99-104 and 136-146

16 Willem F. Daems, Welche Abkürzung gebrauchte Rudolf Steiner in seiner Mistelsaft-Notiz? (Which abbreviation did Rudolf Steiner use in his mistletoe note?) Der Merkurstab (Stuttgart) 41(2) (1988), 136-138; Ill. on p. 136

17 There are various etymological derivations of the German name for Chelidonium. It is easily recognizable that Schöllkraut is derived from Coelidonum. In addition there are derivations based on the old German verb sceljan = schielen (looking cross-eyed) (indication for ophthalmological use), thus Schielkraut, in dialect also Scheelkraut.

18 Thorough historical monographs:

a. Hedwig Schwarz, Pharmaziegeschichtliche Pflanzenstudien. Chelidonium majus L., p. 12-47. Mittenwald 1931

b. Karl Daniel und Dieter Schmaliz, Das Schöllkraut. (Arzneipflanzen in Einzeldarstellungen 1). Stuttgart 1939

19 With the dissertation of Gunster the problems were in priciple already solved: Pieter Engelbertus Gunster, Overzicht van en bijdrage tot de kennis van medicinale Curcuma (temoe lawak) [Overview and a contribution to knowledge of the medical curcuma (Temu Lawak)]. Dissertation, Groningen 1943

20 Hagers Handbuch der Pharmazeutischen Praxis, Ed. P. H. List and L. Hörhammer, Vol. 4 (C-G). Berlin/Heidelberg/New York 1973, p. 386

21 Otto Leeser, Lehrbuch der Homöopathie. Spezieller Teil B/II: Pflanzliche Arzneistoffe. Heidelberg 1971, p. 291f

22 Stictly interpreted, with Rudolf Steiner's recommendation - in summer 1920 - to treat the combination of chelidonium and curcuma "by centrifuging like the mistletoe preparation," a Choleodoron preparation was intended in accordance with Rudolf Steiner's concept.

23 Wilhelm Pelikan, Healing Plants, Vol. I, Chelidonium, Mercury Press, Spring Valley, 1998; Curcuma, in Heilpflanzenkunde, Band II, Dornach[2] 1984, p. 97f

24 Not a single paper on Chelidonium in the relevant literature of phytopharmacology shows what - so surprisingly - really goes on in the root region of this plant. This phenomenal root growth was observed during certain investigations in the Research Laboratory at the Goetheanum. The illustration comes from: Jochen Bockemühl, Entwicklungsweisen des Klatschmohns im Jahreslauf als Hilfen zum Verständnis verwandter Arten. [Modes of development of Papaver somniferum in the course of the year as help in understanding related species.] In: Elemente der Naturwissenschaft, Heft 19/1973, S. 37-56; the illustration on page 50.

I aquired the photo of curcuma during my student days (about 1935)from the Kolonial-Institut, Amsterdam.

25 Theodor Lang, Gurke, Melone, Kürbis. Ihre Treib- und Freilandkultur, nebst einem Anhang: Die zierenden Kürbisgewächse [Cucumber, melon, pumpkin. Their cultivation in greenhouse and free field. With an appendix: The decorative squash plants.] in (Gartenbau-Bibliothek, 19). 76 S., 15 Ill., Berlin 1909

26 Willem F. Daems, Die Rose ist kalt im ersten Grade, trocken im zweiten. [The rose is cold in the first degree, dry in the second.] Beiträge zu einer Erweiterung der Heilkunst nach geisteswissenschaftlichen Erkenntnissen (Stuttgart) 25 (6) (1972), p. 204-211

27 Without source in my notes. I cannot recall from whom or from where the sketch originates.

28 I am grateful to Dr. med. Felix Baur, Basel, for this indication.

29 A. G. Degenaar published without date and place "Case histories and other medical questions discussed with Rudolf Steiner", (English translation in preparation by Mercury Press.): 1. Case Nr. 120, p. 59 2. Arteriosclerosis. Discussion Aug. 11. 1922, p. 83

30 I quote from the superb edition of: Werner Näf und Mathäus Gabathuler, Walahfrid Strabo. Hortulus. Vom Gartenbau. St. Gallen 1942

31 For an orientation concerning the relationship Rudolf Steiner/Paracelsus see my introduction (p. VII XXXVI) to: Elise Wolfram, Die okkulten Ursachen der Krankheiten (Volumen Paramirum des Paracelsus). Dornach, Verlag am Goetheanum [4] 1991 [12]

32 See the Lemma Nikolaus von Polen (Gundolf Keil) in Verfasserlexikon, Bd. VI, Berlin and New York [2] 1987, p. 1128-1133

33 Theophrastus von Hohenheim, called Paracelsus: Sämtliche Werke. 1. Abt. Medizinische, naturwissenschaftliche und philosophische Schriften. Volumes 1-14. Ed. by Karl Sudhoff, München und Berlin 1922-1933. Quoted with Abt., Bd. and page number, e.g. Sudhoff I,3,43

34 For Paracelsus studies the Sudhoff-Ausgabe is still the best. I quote them (in German) word for word. By reading the German aloud it will be easier to understand the meaning of the passages.

34 Sudhoff I,14,49

35 Sudhoff I,1,12

36 Sudhoff I,2,95

37 Sudhoff I,2,193

38 Sudhoff I,13,201

39 Sudhoff I,14,527

40 Sudhoff I,9,649

41 Sudhoff I,2,649

42 Sudhoff I,10,152/3

43 Kurt Goldammer, Der göttliche Magier und die Magierin Natur. Mit Beiträgen zum Magie-Verständnis des Paracelsus (= Kosmosophie, 5). Stuttgart 1991

44 Sudhoff I,14,541

45 Sudhoff I,14,541

46 Sudhoff I,14,542

47 Giovanni Negri, Erbario figurato. Mailand [4]1948, p. 88 (Illustration source)

48 Hans Rutschow attempted in his dissertation Concerning Magnetism in Paracelsus, Cologne, July 26, 1965 [not printed] to deal with this theme exhaustively.

49 Walter Pagel, Paracelsus. An Introduction to Philosophical Medicine in the Era of the Renaissance. Basel, München, Paris [2] 1982 [1958], p. 319

50 The Swabian theologian and theosophist Christoph Friedrich Oetinger (1702-1782) formulated as follows: "The bodies are encompassed by invisible forces ". Cited after: Emil Bock, Boten des Geistes, Stuttgart [4] 1987, p. 86

Chelidonium / Curcuma comp.

Composition:	
Chelidonium majus, Rhizoma and roots	2.4%
Curcuma xanthorrhiza, Rhizoma	9.6%
Curcubita maxima, Pulpa Fructus	79.3%
Excipients	8.7%

Form of Medication: Tablets

Indications: Disorders of bile formation and bile secretion

Use: 1-2 tablets three times daily before meals

Package Sizes: 30 gm, 100gm

Keep away from moisture before use!

Manufacture and Sales: Weleda, Inc. Arlesheim, Switzerland

About the Author

Willem Frans Daems was born on December 3, 1911 in Amsterdam, Holland, he died December 28,1994 in Arlesheim. After graduating from pharmacy school he worked at his trade until Weleda called him to Arlesheim. From September 1955 until his death he was a scientific collaborator there, mostly as a lecturer and writer. He was the editor of Weleda-Korrespondenzblätter for Doctors from 1964 until his death, and from 1967 on he brought out the monthly Weleda-Informations Bulletin.

In 1951 he went back to study at Leiden University. His dissertation there in 1967 got him the Venia legendi for Netherlandistik and medical history of the late Middle Ages, and later a teaching position in medical history at the Institute for Medical History at Würzburg University. He was deeply concerned for the interests of the Anthroposophical medical movement, mainly concentrating on medical and pharmaceutical historical aspects. He has published many books and articles in journals.